Vitamins of Life; Understanding what you need for your benefits

By

Emiliano M Espinoza

Prefix

So you want to become healthy, Great for you! This book will help understand vitamins, calories, water & your body so that you may reach whatever goal you have. If your reading this book & have no clue of foods & health & don't know where to start diet wise, you reading this is an amazing step into your journey & I'm proud of you. Yes you, your body will thank you so much & you should feel great knowing that you will become a better person physically & mentally.

If you've already started on your fitness journey & want to enrich it, I'm also proud of you. You reading this proves nothing will stop you from becoming better & better. Keep up the good work, let nothing hold you back from become more healthy & informed.

If you're well-seasoned, already knowledgable of different foods & just want a re-fresh of what you know or forgotten, then I must say...I'm proud of you.

You made it this far, nothing wrong with a reminder of what to intake & what it is your intaking, you do have a body to maintain. Now, for everyone, this book will *only* explain the vitamins of the human body, what they do, where to get them & how to intake them. At the time of this writing, I am enrolled in the Penn-Foster College for 'Fitness & Nutrition' & have learned quite a lot writing this book & attending online classes. I started going to college for health & fitness because I love working out & making sure I'm healthy. I have a wealth of knowledge & I would love to spread to help those who enjoying improving their health or want to get started doing so. My job, as the author, is to give you this information so that it may *help* you with your decisions. I also want to emphasize that I am NO doctor or physician. If you have health concerns, contact your doctor & speak with them. I am a man that's no different from you; I want to enhance my body, preserve it, love it & take very good care of it. You're going to understand just how vital these vitamins are & how extravagant your body is, it's no wonder we should really be grateful for how our bodies work.

You see, there's a lot of research that was done before & during the writing of this book. If you're like me, you do deep research so that you may fully understand a subject. Well, since I love my body, abide by it's needs & this 'll be the only human body I'll be allowed to have, I have done hours & hours of studying, understanding & being well informed. I was doing so before going to college, during college & will do continue on after college. You may have done the same as me, maybe not to such an extent or even at all. Whatever the case maybe, I went through the loops, forehead rubs & sighs for you, so that I can present to you & spread that knowledge to you. I made this simple & threw in some humor for you, why not enjoy yourself a laugh & have some fun while becoming better?

No, I won't show any meal plans either, but I will show different foods & explain them as well. As I've said, I'm here to help you make decisions. I'll be unbiased on this matter as well, I will not tell what meal plan to take on either or include any of my own beliefs. you get the idea, I don't want to be redundant. I'm to present with you facts of the vitamins, & the body's needs, you will make the adjustments accordingly. With all this being said & understood, I will lead you on to becoming more well informed & wiser with these pages, starting off with water & your blood, then all the vitamins will be listed alphabetically. The other minerals you need'll come after I list off the vitamins. I'll also give you a well thought out insight of all the benefits & drawbacks too. Hey, there is something called 'too much of a good thing' & I'd be leading you astray if I didn't mention the good & bad, I'm serious about giving you this information. I'll also label how each vitamin is consumed & how best to do, whether they're fat-soluble or water-soluble.

Let's begin with the knowledge in the pages & become more intelligent & mentally equipped to take us to a better life with the foods we eat!

Acknowledgements

For Sherrell, your friendship is valued beyond words. To give further inspiration to me, leaves me astonished, speechless & even more blessed, thank you.

For Barry, my fellow guardian on *Destiny,* your alliance is God-given, you're amazing. The laughs never cease between us.

For Avi, I don't even have to explain, but I must. Our bond is stronger than steel & submerged in gold. I don't recall any dull moments with you.

For Ri'chard, the knowledge we exchange & fun we have will always stay with me, you just make sure to do the same.

For Quentaz, I never expected to meet a man of such wisdom & understanding, it's no surprise we just clicked.

For Justin, you got my back & I got yours, your help in the workshop has molded me to become better. I love you like my mother had you.

For Sawyer, the only riddler bigger than me, but a man of acceptance. You made sure I've left smarter in our conversations. Let me tender this one time, lol.

For Toya, you made sure to stand by my side, no matter what. What more could I say, you're awesome.

For JP, you took me under your wing as your little brother, I take heed of the things you've said, even in hard moments.

For Eric, you've respected me just as I was, no need to prove myself. something so simple, yet so big, it allowed us to become a unique duo.

For Jada, you're heart is pure & you never stop being you, & you made sure to stay in contact, that alone is sweet of you.

& I can't forget, my mother & father. I love you two, no matter what, the love'll never flicker away.

Table of contents

CHAPTER 1:

THE IMPORTANCE OF A DIET & EXERCISE

For starters, we have to understand that in order to reap the benefits of these vitamins & be fit with our lives, we have to tack down the concept of a diet. Yes, I know, its a word we all hear, hate & a thing we avoid or we simply cannot stay on top of. It's difficult to be on a diet, I know from experience from myself. No matter what kind of plan you follow, it's difficult to stay on our 'A game'. If you don't struggle with this issue, then that's great news for you & I encourage to persist. If you do however, do not beat yourself down, that's a waste of time & a confidence destroyer, neither things we need. Now, if you look up the definition of a diet from the *Cambridge Dictionary* it'll say: *food,* especially *a course of recommended foods, for losing weight or as a treatment for an illness etc".* or "*to eat certain kinds of foods to lose weight* ". Of course you can follow a diet to gain weight as well, for those interested in doing so.

But to do as I say I would do, I will simplify the already simple definition for you. A diet is a plan of foods that one takes on to obtain whichever goal they may have for their body. What that goal you have for your body, there's a diet for that goal. You find that diet, conjure up your own, whatever the case may be & you stick with it until the end & beyond. That might sound a little intimidating to you, but I promise you this; you will be so proud of yourself for staying on course & focused on that diet. The benefits you'll reap from that diet will be like no other & you'll be astonished by what you can do. No obstacle is too big for you, that much I can tell you!

Exercise has the same concept, you formulate a plan to get yourself in shape & run with it. You get your body moving, staying strong, flexible & mobile. Combine this with a diet & you'll reach that goal, no matter what it takes. You just have to be dedicated & disciplined to do so. With these words ingrained into your mind &

put into action, your health will change dramatically, in which ever direction you choose. You also don't have to do it alone. You get a doctor involved, let them perform various tests on you, get those results & now you can head off in the right direction. Hey, having guidance from a professional doctor is a very big step & clears out the fog that's hiding your goal.

How to obtain your goal

List out your diet & exercise routine. Draw out your map to your goal. Go see a doctor, list out a diet & exercise routine, follow through according to your schedule (things happen in life & you have a life, but a little bit of something is better than nothing, small steps compound) & you'll reach your goal. When you jot down that plan, you can visually see it & be reminded of it to stay true to it! As you move down the list, you'll draw close to your goal.

Be Disciplined. Quitting, anxiety, doubt, these are all common factors on why people neglect their plan & their goal. It's not easy, everyone knows that, but it's not impossible. To be disciplined is the back bone of your plan, the foundation to your goal. If your discipline is weak, you'll only hinder & set yourself back. You will do that, no more. You will stick to that plan, you will reach that. Whatever it is you have to do, you do that. Indulging on that box of cookies is a no go, sitting on that couch feeling bad for yourself or binge watching whatever it is on that phone or tablet is a no go. Do the opposite of those things. Stay eating healthy, stay moving, stay strong.

Study & Engage. Do not just go through the motion of a workout, perform them with proper technique to fully engage in it. Do not just stuff your face with fruit cups & call it day. Follow that diet plan to the fullest. Stay & understand what is your doing, your mind will connect so much better with the equipped & applied knowledge, hence making you more aware of what you're doing, why you're doing it & how to do it.

Desire & Demand that goal. It doesn't matter if you plan these things if you have no motivation to stick to it. You have to want that body & demand it. When I tell you to demand that body, you have to be stern & focused for it, not just simply want. You have to want the goal first, then you have to demand it from yourself. No one else can want or obtain that goal for you. You as a person have to desire

& demand it. No cheat days, no quitting, you have that image in your head, now run after it

Love yourself. You have to be confident & respect yourself. Do not beat yourself down & have negative self talk in any shape or form. That'll ruin the focus & bring down your motivation. Keep your head high, remain resilient & go for the prize.

Heed this words & form your plan for that goal. You have it in you, don't say you don't.

CHAPTER 2:

OUR BLOOD!

To grasp a better understanding the vitamins, foods & water of life & how they benefit us, we first need to understand blood. The blood that flows in our body is so special, so amazing & believe it or not, quite complex! But have no worries, I have you covered. With this fluid flowing in our bodies, its the upmost importance to understand it before we move on, do not skip this chapter (or any chapter, I beg of you).

So what in the world is blood? Well, blood is the fluid that allows our body to work the way it does. The "life force" if you will. The job of our blood is put like this: It carries oxygen throughout the body, takes away carbon dioxide (a waste byproduct your body produces after using food for energy, but still needed), other waste products, transport nutrients into the cells, which is pumped by the heart, running a huge track (your body) & flows back into your heart via blood vessels, repeating the process. With blood transporting nutrients & oxygen into your cells, you get why I want you to know more about blood. It controls your body's temperature, protects you from infections, formulates blood clots to stop bleeding, carries hormones, electrolytes, etc. giving you the ability to function as you do now. Your blood flows through veins, arteries & capillaries.

Your blood is made of four things; red blood cells, white blood cells platelets & plasma. Now these four have very important duties to fulfill, when they fulfill those duties, your body functions as normal & when they don't, that's catastrophic to say the least. Your blood cells are made inside the bone marrow, which is very soft tissue found in the middle of your bones. You can thank bone marrow for making 95% of your blood cells, with some of your organs making & regulating the rest, but we won't get into that part. Your cells start off as stem cells, which in turn, grow & mature into designated jobs, of course, falling underneath the four categories mentioned earlier. They can develop into cells for each organ or muscles, but they all (in general) perform the same jobs.

Blood is a tissue *and* a fluid. As said by Professors C.Lockard Conley & Robert S. Schwartz , "*Blood is both a tissue and a fluid. It is a tissue because it is a collection of similar specialized cells that serve particular functions. These cells are suspended in a liquid matrix (), which makes the blood a fluid.*" That may seem confusing, so let me simplify it. Blood is a tissue because of the specialized cells that serve their own purpose, also being suspended in plasma, making it a fluid. To break down what 'suspended' means in this context, suspended means that something solid is spread in a liquid without dissolving in that liquid. Think of muddy water or flour in water. In this case, the blood cells & plasma. Stay with me, we're diving deeper into the blood.

Your **red blood cells**, aka 'erythrocytes' (hard to pronounce, I know) are what carry oxygen throughout the body with the help of hemoglobin, a iron-rich protein, which also happens to give red blood cells their color. Oxygen is what gives you energy & powers up your cells. They make up 45% of your blood, take up to 7 days to fully mature & have a pretty small life span of 120 days, then these cells are replaced with new ones. It's your red cells that carry the carbon dioxide to your lungs to exhale. When you have low red blood cells, you'll notice you're fatigued, your vision gets all blurry, you'll get headaches, feel dizzy, experience muscle weakness & shortness of breath.

What causes low red blood cells is malnutrition, vitamin deficiencies of iron, B9 ,B12, copper, vitamin A & vitamin C (which'll all be explained later, hold your horses) & pre-existing medical conditions such as sickle cells, cancer, cancer treatments, kidney disease, blood loss & organ failure. We won't get into the details of the pre-existing medical conditions, but it does help to list them. To get your red blood cells back on track, you'll definitely want to consume foods with the mentioned vitamins, & exercise. You see, exercising will increase your heart rate, thus increasing the demand of oxygen from your heart & brain, which in turn'll produced that hemoglobin & combine that with a balanced meal, your bone marrow has what it needs to produce your red blood cells. You'll also want to reduce alcohol consumption, for men, moderate drinking of alcohol is two or less & for women, its one or less.

What causes high red blood cells is smoking, living in high altitudes, taking anabolic steroids (erythropoietin for one example), hell, even stress. Throw in dehydration in the mix as well. Some medical conditions such as kidney tumors, hypoxia, sleep apnea, carbon monoxide exposure (with smoking being the most common issue) & Polycythemia vera, which is a rare cancer that makes the bone marrow produce too many red blood cells. You'll feel some of the same symptoms of of having low red blood cells, but with you'll also experience joint pain, itchy skin, nose bleeds, numbness/tingling & a decrease in blood flow. Now, keep in mind, a person may not experience any symptoms for either low or high RBC, so it's a great idea to check in with your doctor.

To lower your risk of high red blood cells, you have to quit smoking, which I know, is easier said than done. You also want to intake some vitamin B12 reduce your iron intake. I know I mentioned the importance of iron beforehand, everything has to be balanced. Exercise to keep improve heart & lung functionality & drink plenty of water, fall back on the red meats too. Having high RBC doesn't mean you have a medical condition, you can fix one cause by drinking water when dehydrated, the plasma is decreased, which increase red blood cell concentration. As I said, speak to your doctor

Your **white blood cells**, medical term 'leukocytes' makes up less than 1% of your blood, but still plays a colossal-size role, because these cells are apart of your immune system. When bacteria, fungi, viruses etc. become an issue to your body, their job is to go against those guys, fend them off & destroy them. Your white blood cells are divided into 5 segments that specialize in against various infections. You got:

Neutrophils- destroys bacteria & fungi, is the largest group of white blood cells & is your first line of defense. They also have to shortest life span of the bunch, of less than a day, so the bone marrow keeps them coming.

Monocytes- destroys viruses, bacteria, protozoa & removes damaged/bad cells. They also have a longer life span.

Basophils- these guys react to allergens & lets everyone else know there's an invader in your blood stream

Eosinophils- They assist the basophils with allergic responses & kill parasites & cancerous cells.

Lymphocytes- Produce the antibodies you need to fight against infections

What can weaken the immune system & cause fluctuating levels of white blood cell count are infections, because your body has to produce more to fend them off, HIV/AIDS, chemotherapy & even some medicines. There are foods to help your immune system such as yogurts & garlic.

Moving on to your **platelets** or 'thrombocytes', they'll be the first to respond when blood vessels are damaged & when you're bleeding. They repair damaged blood vessels. When they're non-active, they're shaped like plates, hence their name. These platelets stop you from bleeding by forming blood clots, stretching tentacles from themselves. This maneuver allows the cells to flow by them as they do their job. Platelets are the lightest part of your body & account for less than 1% of your blood, same as white blood cells. However, there are thousands of these platelets in a single drop of blood. Drinking too much alcohol will reduce these platelet though.

Finally, your **plasma**, where the cells & platelets linger within. Plasma makes up 55% of your blood & helps clot your blood, give waste to your lungs, liver & kidney to get rid of them, maintains your blood pressure, blood circulation & maintains body temperature by releasing or taking heat. Plasma also takes hormones, proteins, & nutrients to parts of the body that needs it. This is why during blood drives, plasma is so sought after, because it provides so many benefits. Plasma itself is 92% water & 7% protein.

Now you see why I broke down blood & what it is, what it does, & why we need it? Without blood, we'd be dead in minutes. The things we put into our body will affect our blood, & since we now understand blood a little better, even with a small glimpse, you begin to more cognitive of what you consume. That's good, we want to make wiser decisions for our bodies, just look at the functions & roles of blood alone. Before we continue on, we never did discuss carbon dioxide.

Carbon dioxide is a gas found in the body. When your cells convert sugar & fats into energy (the foods you eat) it then creates carbon dioxide. 90% of the carbon dioxide in your body is bicarbonate, while the rest of it just dissolves in your blood or is found to be carbonic acid. *Dr. Matthew Eng,* who has his credentials from the University of Hawaii & the University of Washington, explains that *"CO2, [carbon dioxide] especially in the form of bicarbonate, plays an important role in maintaining the pH of the blood. Bicarbonate acts as a buffer, preventing blood from becoming too acidic or basic".* In short, carbon dioxide maintains blood pH balance & controls your breathing.

CHAPTER 3:

THE WATER WE NEED

We understand blood now, a little better. Really, a whole lot better, we'll do the same thing for water. You hear it all the time, how important water is for us as humans, how much to drink, when to drink, how to drink it, where to get it, who sales the best, it all gets overwhelming at times! Yet it seems most people don't truly understand water, just get their heads crammed with different products of water, whose the best or what not. People get these expensive water bottles, huge jugs to store water, it's a damn fiasco. Nope, no advertisements this time, this is strictly about water itself & only water, why it's needed & what to do with it. I'm here to inform, not pitch a sale for any these corporates.

How We Benefit From Water

Everything that breathes, eats, moves, sleeps, poops & annoys you must have water to continue its life. Where you find water, is where you find life. Get this, did you know 97% of water on our planet is salt? That leaves 3% for us to consume, puts things into perspective doesn't it? It has no taste, no color, but still the most important liquid of Earth & the Universe. We're not talking about space though, let's bring things down a gazillion notches to us humans.

What water does for our bodies, is that it carries the vitamins & minerals to our cells & removes waste from our cells, which means it's aiding our digestion system & creates something known as hydrochloric acid. Your stomach creates hydrochloric acid, & it breaks down protein for you, with the help of pepsinogen & when these two meet up, they form an enzyme called pepsin. Since our bodies can't break down entire proteins, pepsin turns proteins into amino acids, making them absorbable. Protein isn't the only thing hydrochloric acid works with, but we won't steer off topic. Don't worry yourself either, hydrochloric acid, in combination with some potassium chloride & sodium chloride, your stomach acid as a pH level of 1-2. That's pretty dang low if you ask me, but your body is set up to protect your stomach's lining from being eaten all up. Just some facts to throw in, moving on.

Water is also a very powerful lubricant for our joints, thus allowing the production of something called synovial fluid. This fluid greatly reduces friction between our joints, like your elbow, knees, wrists, hips & your shoulders. When you drink water, it allows bloods' volume, viscosity & circulation to be right where they need to be, so that you may function as a human. Water'll maintain cell shape as well, along with protecting your brain & spinal cord.

I already know you heard of the general rule of thumb of 8 cups of water of day'll keep you up & running, but that's too outdated & research has shown that our requirements vary from person to person. Many experts'll tell you that everyone's needs is different, how much water you're brother will need is going to be whole lot different from you & even you best friend's. However over at the *Harvard Health Publishing & Medical school,* they give healthy adult men an average of 15.5 cups a day & for healthy women an average of 11.5 cups a day. Now notice I said "healthy adults" & "average". Now also notice I said that everyone is different. How exactly is everyone different? Your medical conditions, your age, gender, how active you are & just your overall health all play a factor in how much your water your body will need. For your children who run around all day, *Children's health* has an explanation for them, based on age & gender. For both boys & girls aged 1-8, they'll need about 4 cups a day. For boys aged 9-13, that goes up to 8 cups a day, aged 14-18, that number becomes 11 cups per day. For girls aged 9-13, it's 7 cups per day & 14-18, 8 cups per day. 1 cup is 8 fl oz, so to get an exact measurement for yourself, multiply the cup by 8. So 2 cups'll be 16 oz, 3 cups'll be 24 oz etc. Now this rule only applies to those that weigh up to 100 lbs, drink about half of your weight, so 80 lbs will need about 40 oz. As I stated for adults, this is average for children. Whatever health factors or outside forces may be going on will change that number for them. To get the most accurate number for yourself & children, speak to a doctor & let them give you the real answer.

The Ugly side of water (too much or too little)

Your kidneys do a great job filtering out water & releasing it as urine. Your kidneys make all of the adjustments responding to water levels with the help of a hormone called the 'arginine vasopressin' which is released when water balances is changing, all done within 40 seconds. To help you visualize that, the reason you urinate immediately after drinking more than what you need is because your over-hydrated or your urination is put on hold to keep water within when dehydrated. Listen to your body, my friends.

When your dehydrated or lack water, you're losing more fluid than what you're taking in, what'll happen is that your kidney'll start to fail, because it's strained, it can't release waste, forming kidney stones (no fun), you'll have seizures because if the electrolytes aren't right, which carries electric pulses in your cells to regulate the water in your body, your muscles will contract on their own & you'll lose consciousness. Your brain can also swell up because you when begin to drink again, your body is going to pull way too much fluid into cells, making them rupture & if *that* happens to your brain cells, that'll be fatal. You can combat mild or moderate dehydration with no issues, but anything severe, will require immediate attention. Causes of dehydration is lack of water, hot weather, extreme diarrhea & extreme workouts. Let's keep our selves hydrated, for our sakes.

Now on the same token, there is a thing called over-hydration. Yes, it is possible & yes, it is fatal. Over-hydration occurs when you drink too much water or your kidney retains too much water. This'll lead to something called water poisoning or toxicity & cause an imbalance in electrolytes, making them diluted. Sodium becomes diluted, leading to hyponatremia. Sodium controls how much water goes in & around your cells, but when sodium is reduced, water will rush into your cells, leading to inflammation & ruptures of the cells, which includes your brain too. Signs of over-hydration will be nausea, confusion, a headache & colorless urine, you want a nice pale yellow in your urine. Let's fall back on hydration as well, got to found that balance.

To summarize everything on everything you just read, the best way to prevent any bad thing happening to you & is to drink in moderation & listen to your body depending on conditions. If you're drinking too much, you'll know it, if you're drinking too little, you'll know it. Don't ignore these signs trying to become a a health guru, it'll back fire & you'll be flustered. You'll find that sweet spot yourself or through your doctor.

CHAPTER 4:

CLASSIFICATION OF VITAMINS

Our vitamins are split into two groups, known as water-soluble or fat soluble. That means each vitamin is better absorbed either through the fats in our body or through the water we consume. I'll be sure to let you know how each vitamin is taken & where to get it from, I'll even label them for you. But exactly are vitamins? Vitamins are a form of nutrients found in the foods that we eat that are very essential for our health, growth & the function of our bodies & organs.

Fat-Soluble

Fat-soluble cells cannot dissolve in water, whatsoever., they dissolve in fats & oils. They're stored in our fatty tissues, known as adipose & in our livers. They're absorbed by fat globules, travel through our small intestines & gets put in our blood stream. With that being said, these vitamins are best taken with fats in our foods, healthy fats that is of course. Vegetable oils, olive oil, greek yogurt, peanut butter & seeds have these healthy fats. These vitamins are also known as non-essential vitamins because our bodies synthesize them. To translate that for you, synthesize means to 'produce a substance by a chemical reaction in the human body'. Do not be mistaken though, your body'll still need these vitamins, make to sure get them in. There are just four fat-soluble vitamins, which include vitamins A, D, E & K & stay inside your body longer. Everyone else is water-soluble.

The Categories of fats

Now there are four types of fats: Monounsaturated, polyunsaturated, saturated & trans fat. The trans fat & saturated are the fats you want to stay away from.

Trans fats are found in highly processed foods such as packaged foods, fast food, fried food & processed breads. Trans fats are artificially made through a process called hydrogenation, which Harvard explains that "is used to turn healthy oils into solids and to prevent them from becoming rancid." It lowers your good cholesterol (which builds healthy cells), causes heart disease, strokes & weight gain to list a few. Your body literally doesn't need trans fat, so kick it out of your life, its even been banned in the U.S. as well as of 2015!

You'll want to limit the intake of saturated fats,& there's a huge grey area concerning saturated fats. Yes, you'll need it, but at small dosages, since they raise cholesterol & cause arteries to get blocked up in your heart, thus increasing the chance for strokes & heart attacks. But it's been shown to lower triglyceride levels, when these levels are up, up & away, they increase your chance of heart disease. That leaves saturated fats to be more neutral than bad some experts would argue. But there still hasn't been any proof of health benefits from it either, so no one can call out a dietary change really. With that being said, limit your consumption of saturated fats which can be found in meats, cheese, milk, & yogurt to list a few & go for the other two fats. Yeah, saturated fat is kind of confusion, but still needed, at a limit though. You only need about 22 grams of saturated fats per day.

Monounsaturated fat makes up 97% of the fat in your body, along with saturated. It lowers your cholesterol, protects against heart disease, improve insulin sensitivity, strengthen your bones & even manage your weight. That's a lot of good coming from monounsaturated fat. Hell, get this, it's shown to allow the absorption of calcium into your bones through animal research too, giving more density. who wouldn't want strong bones? You'll want 22-44 grams of this stuff to be healthy

Polyunsaturated fat is actually split into two types, omega-6 & omega-3 fatty acids. What this fat does is lower inflammation, decrease blood pressure & give you that good cholesterol. Oh, the benefits don't stop there, this fat is even found in the brain, aiding in gene expression, cell growth, kicking that depression to the curb & help people who are bi-polar. You want better sleep, get some Polyunsaturated fat in you to do just that, with tests conducted by *The University of Missouri-Kansas City School of Medicine,* they found by using patients & testing their sleep with their diets in mind, *"that that disordered membrane fatty acid patterns may play a causal role in OSA...".* (OSA being Obstructive Sleep Apnea). Even with this study, there's still research on this to be done. It reduces menstrual pain for you & is way more effective than ibuprofen will ever be. Get some food & avoid OTC medicines; win-win. For people with glacier-thick glasses on their face (me included), your vision'll improve too & prevent macular degeneration, which causes vision loss. It helps with the functionality of the photoreceptor cells (the guys that detect light & color for you). in the retina. This heaven-sent fat can be found in almonds, salmon, pecans etc. Doctors recommend to take one-two servings of 2.5 ounces of fatty fish per week.

Note: All intake recommendations based on the 2,000 calorie diet, speak with your doctor for more help.

Water-Soluble

Water soluble vitamins dissolve in the water in our bodies, gets absorbed in our tissues & are used immediately. That means you got to keep these vitamins coming in through your diet, your body won't store them & can't make them on its own or in other words, these vitamins aren't synthesized, making them known as 'essential vitamins'. Vitamin C & all vitamin B's (yes, there are multiple B's for you to take) are absorbed through water & gets released through your urine right after, except for B12, that sticks around in your liver for years to come. You can get these vitamins from oranges, kiwis, black beans etc. & be good to go.

CHAPTER 5:

VITAMIN A (FAT-SOLUBLE)

Finally, we can get started with the vitamins! After everything you just read previously, you can now plan your meals a little better or take your vitamins a lot wiser than before you opened these pages (seriously, that information is definitely going to help you out!), just like we had a very brief discussion of intakes on fat, I'll obviously be doing the same here. Without further ado, lets begin.

What is vitamin A (retinol)

According to the *National Institutes of Health* or the 'NIH' for the sake of memory, vitamin 'A' is the name given to a group of chemicals which are called 'retinoids' or chemicals that derive from vitamin 'A' & from their website, it states that vitamin A is *"...involved in immune function, cellular communication, growth and development, and male and female reproduction."*. That's the bare minimum of what it is, we have to go further than that. Vitamin 'A' helps form & allows the heart, lungs, liver & the other organs stuffed inside of your body to work properly. Not only does it help with sexual reproduction systems & your immune system, it also helps with your bones being able to grow & your vision allowing you to see. Vitamin A allows the production & growth of your white blood cells, strengthens your bones, teeth & makes your skin a whole lot healthier as well.

Vitamin A is also an anti-oxidant, which is a substance that'll prevent or delay the damage of cells. We have two forms of vitamin A, one known as 'Performed vitamin A', which come from animal products, fortified foods & vitamin supplements. The other one being known as 'Provitamin A carotenoids', which is found naturally in plant foods.

Benefits of vitamin A

Eye Health- We got some nice things to get from vitamin A. One being it strengthens & helps your eyes from night blindness, called 'nyctalopia'. Now this doesn't affect the ability to see during the day or in well lit areas, but solely the night. How this is happens is that when you're deprived of vitamin A, there's a important thing in your eyes called the 'rhodopsin' & is very sensitive to light, won't have the ability to adjust to darker areas or the night. Please note, nyctalopia is not a disease itself, but its an underlying condition to a eye disease, to treat it, you'll have to found the issue & go accordingly. We won't dive into that, but to rid of this issue, is to increase vitamin A intake. Vitamin A also helps with general health of your eyes, it'll help slow the process of blindness in older adults.

Immune System- Vitamin A gives power to your immune system, with it being tied to the production & function of your white blood cells & supports the mucous membranes in your body as well, which catches the bacteria from infecting your body.

Skin- Vitamin A helps your skin to glow & look luscious too, who wouldn't want that for themselves? How it does that is by reducing build up of dead skin cells & oil in your skin glands, which get clogged up, giving you the inflammation on your skin, giving you the worst thing in whole wide world; acne! Vitamin A sweeps that away from you, while at the same making your skin glow brighter & make your skin tone more vibrant.

Bones- Vitamin D, calcium & protein get all the praise for helping your bones, but what about vitamin A? Vitamin A prevents your bones from fracturing as easily, but there's still plenty of research needed to confirm how & why this is.

Reproduction- For men & women, this vitamin is essential for reproduction & the genitals. For men, this vitamin helps maintain sperm health count, & the penile tract. For women, this vitamin makes sure the eggs are in good shape & allows them to mature properly. It also improves quality of cervical fluid, in turn making the sperm in contact help live longer & help fertilize better. During pregnancy, it'll help the unborn baby have a better skeleton, nervous system heart, eyes & pancreas.

Drawbacks; Too many!

Too much of anything, is not a good thing & that includes vitamins & minerals. If you have too much vitamin A, you'll feel nauseas, dizziness & even become sensitive to sunlight & have blurry vision. Oh, & those health benefits for your baby? Those can quickly turn into birth defects, especially synthetic formats of vitamin A (we'll talk about this soon, hang tight). The best way to avoid this list of no-good things is to get your vitamins from a balanced diet & especially from plants. Hell, too much vitamin A can interfere with vitamin D, we want everything to be harmonious & working together!

Too Little

If you have too little of vitamin A, you'll experience nyctalopia (as we previously mentioned), can cause white patches on your eyes & can even experience something else called 'Xerophthalmia'! Xerophthalmia is when your eyes are very dry & if you don't get this treated, it can lead to night blindness & even permanent blindness. Your skin becomes dry, along with your hair as well & you'll be more prone to infections. You'll experience infertility & be more fatigued.

How to get Vitamin A

The best way to get your vitamins is through a balanced diet, no matter what. Here, we have a list of foods you can get this vitamin & believe it or not, there are two types of vitamin A; one we call preformed vitamin A & the other we call provitamin A. Preformed vitamin A is from meat products, while provitamin comes from plants. Preformed vitamin A is the active version, your body uses it just as it comes. Provitamin A is considered an inactive type & used by your body to make vitamin A & has something called 'beta-carotene' that gives the fruits & veggies the deep, bright colors they have.

Also, from the *University of Rochester Medical Center* you may be surprised that they state the following: "*The vitamin A your body makes from beta-carotene doesn't build up in your body to toxic levels. But vitamin A from animal sources can.*" Now wait just a minute, because they still provide a warning as well, stating: "*Beta-carotene doesn't seem to be toxic in large doses. But high doses over a long time can lead to carotenemia. This causes your skin to become yellowish orange.*" So eating this over time in high doses will give you problems. This is why I emphasize on a balanced diet, everything has to be in moderation for it to work out. The synthetic version of vitamin A is the main (but not only) culprit of birth defects, it's way better to get your vitamins from foods. Here are a list of foods, both animal & plant, to receive this amazing vitamin:

Beef liver, lamb liver, salmon, bluefin tuna, goat cheese, cheddar cheese, eggs, oysters, red peppers, collard, carrots, spinach, red peppers, mango, grapefruit, tangerine & passion fruit to list some. Remember, a balanced diet people, not too many, not too little.

Speak with your healthcare provider for details on a diet

CHAPTER 6:

VITAMINS B1-B5 (WATER-SOLUBLE)

What is Vitamin B?

There's a whole bunch of vitamin B's out there, we'll break them down & see how they help us out as humans. In essence & to summarize Vitamin B, its a vitamin that converts our foods into energy for our bodies & they act as coenzymes; all of them fall under this. A coenzyme activates or gives assistant to the enzymes in your body to start up chemical reactions, they don't operate on their own & need enzymes to start working. What the heck is an Enzyme? Those are little things that speed up the process of chemical reactions in our bodies. Each of the eight vitamin B's have different ways of powering up our enzymes. It goes like this; B1, B2, B3, B5, B6, B7, B9, & B12. There is no B4, B8, B10 or B11, as they are no longer considered vitamins. Obviously they have their own names as well, & if you ever want to take them all at once, that's where B-Complex comes into the picture, as supplements of course. Let's discuss each of the B's we have, we might as well! Now because we have a crowd of vitamin B, we'll list each one & group the benefits, drawbacks & where to find them as one big thing, we're still going to separate them, so read closely. We're doing vitamins B1-B5 first.

Vitamin B1, Thiamine (pronounced Thia-mean)

This vitamin is responsible for the growth, functionality & the development of our organs. It also makes our nerves function correctly & makes sure our bodies use carbohydrates in the correct manner as well. Really important stuff here as you can see! If you don't get enough of B1/Thiamine, you'll lose your appetite, become more confused, have a foggy mind & in severe cases, you can experience nerve damage, with your muscles being weaken & tingling all over. Its not often for people to be thiamine deficit, but people who struggle with alcoholism, Crohn disease or kidney dialysis are more prone to these issues.

Beriberi is a disease that stems from the lack of vitamin B1, which, according to the *Mount Sinai* website, *"...loss of mental alertness, difficulty breathing, and heart damage..."* . Now get this, vitamin B is considered safe & non-toxic, even when taken in high amounts but can still cause you to be drowsy & have relaxed muscles. Still, be careful. You can find vitamin B1 in these foods for example: Pork, eggs, black beans, oranges, asparagus, cauliflower & trout just to name a few.

Vitamin B2, Riboflavin (Ri-bo-flay-vin)

Moving on to vitamin B2, also know as Riboflavin, this vitamin is responsible for breaking down fats, proteins, carbs & making sure you have steady supply of energy. It turns carbs into a molecule known as adenosine triphosphate (ATP to save our tongues here) & this molecule comes from the food we eat, produces our energy & stores energy in our muscles. It helps to prevent migraines from developing (who doesn't hate those?) & just like vitamin A, can protect your eyes from blindness issues, such as cataracts. That's not all, vitamin B2 helps with the absorption with iron too, preventing anemia in the long run.

If you don't get enough of B2, you'll experience dry skin, cracked lips, eye sensitivity, swollen tongue or throat & even anemia. If you're pregnant, you can develop something called preeclampsia, which is high blood pressure that'll result into eclampsia, causing seizures. *Please note, there are other factors into preeclampsia & eclampsia, speak with your doctor over any concerns while pregnant.*

Just like B1, vitamin B2 hasn't shown any negative side effects of high consumption, but still take caution, especially since the body does NOT store riboflavin. You can find this vitamin in these foods; Almonds, salmon, beef, pork, chicken breast, yogurt, cheese, spinach, fortified oats and cereal & clams.

Vitamin B3, Niacin

Vitamin B3 does the same thing as B2, it makes sure your body has energy derived from the food you eat. However, it does so in its own way. This vitamin splits into three ways; nicotinic acid or niacin (duh..), nicotinamide riboside & nicotinamide. Nicotinamide *riboside* is the synthetic form of niacin (supplement), while nicotinic acid & nicotinamide are natural & can be found in our diets & in supplements.

When you take vitamin B3 as a supplement, your body changes it into 'Nicotinamide Adenine Dinucleotide' or NAD. This coenzyme helps with aging, metabolism & the functionality of the cells. It activates proteins that allow you to have improved memory, strength & combats against weight gain.

These forms are all found in the foods we eat & in supplements. B3 also helps with the regulation of your blood pressure by lowering it, your cholesterol, makes sure you have healthy skin & hair by stopping you from losing moisture & delays your skin from aging as well. It'll also make sure you have yourself a healthy functioning brain & protects your brain & nerves by improving the metabolic processes within your body. This vitamin can also help you with anxiety & depression. It even helps with bone joint flexibility & helps out with inflammation reduction.

If you don't get enough of B3, you can develop a disease known as 'Pellagra' & this disease has "four D's" that is associated with it; Diarrhea, dermatitis (your skin being irritated), dementia & death. Pellagra has symptoms of diarrhea, insomnia, fatigue & even suicidal behavior. In the United States, vitamin B3 is pretty abundant in the foods we eat, so it's more rare, but you can still experience these conditions if you don't get that B3 in you.

If you take in too much B3, you'll undergo something called "Niacin flush" which isn't deadly, but causes great discomfort. Your skin'll become red, you'll become dizzy, blood pressure'll fluctuate & experience itching. You can find this vitamin in these foods; Peanut butter, tuna, chicken liver, chicken breasts, mushrooms, cereals.

Vitamin B5, Pantothenic Acid

Moving onwards to vitamin B5, also called pantothenic acid, is another essential vitamin that works the same way as the other vitamins do. the root word 'Panto' in Greek means "everywhere" so you can found this vitamin..everywhere! B5 helps with the production of red blood cells, makes sure your nervous & digestive system check out green & can help with skin & hair even. Vitamin B5's job is to produce coenzyme A, which turns carbs, fats & protein into energy. Are you noticing a pattern here? I sure am. Anyways, coenzyme A also helps with a neurotransmitter called '*acetylcholine*' which makes it possible for brain cells & nerve cells to communicate with each other, allowing your mental brain & mobility to be possible as it is. This vitamin is also responsible for the production of melatonin, the stuff that makes you have a good nights' rest, something we all need, in all seriousness. For those with eczema (such as myself), this vitamin helps with itch relief, bug bites & can help you combat acne. It can even help you with your depression & anxiety, while boosting your immune system.

If you don't get enough B5 (just like B3, is rare in the United Stated due to abundance) you'll experience fatigue, weakness in your body, pain in your feet, skin issues, insomnia, even muscle contractions. Obviously these issues are unwanted in any capacity, needless to say.

You get too much, you'll be dealing with diarrhea, nausea & heartburn. These are uncomfortable to deal with. You can found this vitamin in the following foods: Mushrooms, sweet potatoes, non-fat greek yogurt, nuts, broccoli, chickpeas & ground beef.

CHAPTER 7:

VITAMINS B6-B12 (WATER-SOLUBLE)

Okay, we're almost done with B vitamin family, we still have a lot of good information to get & we're getting to them. We're going to start off with B6 & continue on the same way we did the other ones.

Vitamin B6, Pyridoxine

Vitamin B6 is like the other vitamins; I feel it's safe to assume there's no need to repeat that anymore, honestly. But we have to, believe me, we do, especially since each one has its own unique characteristics. Vitamin B6 scientific name is Pyridoxine, it helps with the development of your brain, especially your neurotransmitters, helps with the development of red blood cells & boosts your immune system! The neurotransmitters this vitamin is responsible for is the serotonin & dopamine & far less commonly known transmitter, gamma aminobutyric acid (byoo-tir-ik)or GABA for short. All three of these regulate our emotions for us. We're all familiar with serotonin & dopamine, but for those that feel left out by that statement, serotonin maintains your mood (known as the "happy" neurotransmitter), helps with memory, your sleep & libido. Dopamine supports the things listed for serotonin as well, & can affect our learning, attention & our ability to take in pain. Some big things from these transmitters. GABA, the lesser known one sitting in the corner facing the wall, has a pretty big responsibility as well. It prevents your nervous system from being overwhelmed with information by blocking certain brain signals, thus decreasing neuron activity. In return of doing this, it helps out with anxiety, stress & even fear.

If you don't receive enough vitamin B6, you'll experience a few things, one of them being something called 'glossitis'. Glossitis is when your tongue becomes inflamed, then it gets all tender, becomes red, looks smooth & glossy. Of course, a difficulty to speak will arise, too. Another thing that can arise is 'Cheilosis' (ky-loh-sis), that's when your lips become crusty, cracked & start scaling at their ends. Cheilosis usually burns, itches & is painful. Now a lack of B6 isn't the only thing that'll cause this, B9 & B2 deficiency can also cause this. Please understand as well, vitamin deficiencies are NOT the only causes of these issue or any other issue to be listed, but they are one of many root causes, just wanted to throw that out there. Back to B6, without enough of this vitamin, you can also experience seizures & depression.

If you take in too much B6 (these affects come from the supplements mostly, but not limited to), you can actually go through 'sensory ataxia', which is when you lose control of your muscles & your coordination. You'll also have to deal with muscle weakness, twitching & numbness that'll spread throughout the body. Lastly, you can damage your nerves, a condition known as 'neuropathy'. You can find B6 in these foods; Salmon, turkey, rice, waffles, onions, chicken breast, bananas & potatoes.

Vitamin B7, Biotin

Here's a more known vitamin, not known as B7, but by its scientific name, biotin. Why is that you may ask? I'll explain why, vitamin B7 encourages the strengthening of hair & nails(sound familiar now?) & encourages the growth of cells & is very important for your metabolism, playing the role of a coenzyme (here we go with that word again) for fats, carbs & protein. It lowers the blood glucose of those with diabetes by increasing the production of insulin in the pancreas. B7 can also combat neuropathy by reducing nerve damage, but further research is required to really confirm this. However, high dosage of this vitamin has shown to reduce problems with MS (multiple sclerosis) which affects the nervous system, the spinal cord & the brain. Of course, its said to help out with bitter nails, skin & damaged hair, thus the reason why its used so much in hair products & other beauty supplies. Keep in mind, more research is needed to back up these claims, even with some evidence.

If you have a B7 deficiency, you can run into problems such as alopecia, loss of energy, experience seizures, believe or not, hallucinations & depression to list a few.

There isn't much evidence providing too much B7 being an issue, even in high dosages! But, the FDA has suggested to avoid high dosage of B7 if you're preparing for lab testing within three days so that you don't disrupt or affect lab results, since high dosages have shown to interfere with other supplements.

You can find this vitamin in the following foods: Mushrooms, bananas, avocados, sweet potatoes, pink salmon, strawberries & basil.

Vitamin B9, Folate

Vitamin B9 works like the other vitamin B's & this vitamin is useful for a healthy liver, skin & eyes. If you're pregnant or planning to be, this vitamin'll be one of your best friends, we'll dive into why that is. To start off, do NOT mix up 'folate' with 'folic acid'. Its very easy to do so & these words are often substituted for one another, but there differences amongst them. Folate is the natural form of B9, folic acid is the *synthetic* form. Still the same, no doubt, but we have to point that out, especially since your body has to convert folic acid into folate if it's to be used for nutritional gain. We have one more type of B9 called Methylfolate or 5-MTHF, which is natural, easier to digest & can be used immediately by the body. Vitamin B9 creates & fixes your DNA, produce some proteins & supports the maturity of red blood cells. Folic acid can slow down the progression of hearing loss & improve your memory. Folate can improve your heart health by supporting your arteries to remain healthy. For pregnancy, B9 helps with preventing birth defects such as spinal & brain issues & can lower the chances of the baby being born autism & having speech impediment issues . On top of that, it can lower the chance of pre-eclampsia developing for the baby. Vitamin B9 can assist with depression, since studies have shown that low B9 levels is associated with it.

If you're experiencing B9 deficiency, you'll have irregular heartbeats, have a hard time focusing, you can experience hair loss & you can even have mouth sores! If you don't know what mouth sores are, they're real painful sores that'll appear on the tongue, lips, cheeks & the roof of your mouth. They're NOT a pretty sight & you'll have a hard time eating & drinking.

If you're taking in a lot of B9, there really isn't much to worry about, except for one thing; high dosages can actually hide a deficiency of B12! Yes, you read that correctly, too much B9 can actually prevent you from knowing if you have a B12 deficiency & that's not a good thing at all. Keep on reading to learn what these issues can be for B12.

The foods you can find high volumes of B9: Asparagus, beets, citrus fruits, papayas, bananas, walnuts, flaxseeds, beef liver & tomato juice.

Vitamin B12 Cobalamin

The final B vitamin on our list, vitamin B12. We came a long way already, B12 is going to finish us off with more facts for us. B12 is so similar to B9, it helps with the formation & maturity of red blood cells, your DNA, helps with your skin, hair, nails, bones, your mood & memory! B12 is apart of the production for serotonin & has been known to improve your mood because of this. You'll have a lower chance of developing an eye disease called 'Macular Degeneration', which affects the part of the eye known as the macula. The macula is what allows you to see finer details within the retina, when you have macular degeneration, your vision becomes blurry & there's no cure for this disease. Just like B9, if you have low levels of B12, it can really cause depression as well (told you, similar to B9). Vitamin B12 can prevent megaloblastic anemia too, which, according to *healthline.com,* is when *"your body doesn't have enough red blood cells to transport oxygen to your vital organs. This can cause symptoms like fatigue and weakness."* We already discussed the importance of our red blood cells (blood in general) & how the hemoglobin that's found in the red blood cells, is what carries the oxygen throughout the body. Go back to read up on it if need be. For megaloblastic anemia, your red cells are strangely shaped & large, making it difficult to carry oxygen.

A deficiency in vitamin B12 will allow an amino acid called homocysteine to increase dramatically. Homocysteine is split into two substances that allow protein to be created & lowers the level of inflammation in the body & increase the health of your liver. You probably just read that & now thinking "Well why would I want to reduce that?" I'll tell you why. A high level of homocysteine will damage your arteries, which carries oxygen rich cells through the cells & can cause your blood vessels to be blocked up. This'll lead to heart disease & strokes. You also develop dementia. Plenty of B9

& B6 will help balance this out too. A deficiency in B12 will also cause you to feel fatigued, make your skin pale, experience some serious migraines, impair your ability to concentrate since it helps out with your central nervous system & cause muscle cramps. For men, a deficiency can cause ED or erectile dysfunction, due to increased levels of homocysteine.

For high volumes of B12, you really don't have too much to worry about, as long its through food. Taking supplements or injections is where the problems start. If you plan on taking this vitamin through these methods, be aware that you can develop acne & experience kidney failure if you're diabetic. If pregnant, high dosage of this vitamin via supplements/injections can increase the chance of autism in the baby. Rosacea (roe-zay-she-uh) will be an issue for you, which is when your skin flares up on your face, causing redness, swelling & blood vessels to be visible.

You can find high levels of vitamin B12 in the following foods: Lamb, beef, salmon, clam, tuna & milk.

CHAPTER 8:

VITAMIN C (WATER-SOLUBLE)

What is Vitamin C? (Ascorbic Acid)

Alright, now what is vitamin C? It forms your blood vessels, muscles & collagen inside your body & is extremely important to your healing process & protects against something called free radicals. Collagen is the most copious protein in your body, making up 30% of the protein in your body & it gives strength to muscles, skin, bones, tendons & your ligaments. Free radicals are molecules made from your body when it breaks down food, exposed to smoke, the radiation emitting from the sun or tanning bed. These molecules are odd-numbered electrons, making them to uncontrollable & in turn take electrons from the healthy cells in your body, causing them harm & creating health issues for you. We'll get more into the benefits of vitamin C.

Benefits of Vitamin C

Protection against free radicals: As aforementioned above, we already discussed a bit about free radicals & what they do to the body. When these guys are inside your body, they create something known as oxidative stress. Oxidative stress is when there is an imbalance of the free radicals & antioxidants within the body, & occurs naturally & is apart of aging. However, external activities as the ones already stated, expedite this process. Your body creates free radicals within the metabolic process but also creates the antioxidants to balance everything out for you. When these free radicals run rampant, especially for a long period of time, they cause a lot of problems for you. One problem is they'll destroy healthy brain cells & alter other molecules for the brain, leading down the road to Parkinson's disease & Alzheimers. They even damage your DNA structure. They cause your skin to become more wrinkled &

create sun spots. Vitamin C is a huge antioxidant friend of yours, so it'll help prevent all of these issues (not limited to, though).

Supports Iron absorption: Iron is a mineral that helps out with the prevention of anemia, which is when you body has a low number of red blood cells, which in turn prevents you from getting the oxygen you need throughout your body, making you fatigued, cold & giving you pretty bad headaches. Anemia causes muscle weakness due to lack of oxygen, making them less elastic. Iron carries is a big carrier of oxygen for you & can improve your sleep. Iron also gives strength to your immune system, making healing a lot easier for you. Vitamin C improves the body's ability to absorb this mineral.

Strengthens Immune System: While iron improves your immune system through the red blood cells, Vitamin C itself helps with the production of white blood cells (check back to blood chapter for memory refreshment if need be) & gives those cells protection from free radicals & other damaging molecules you'll encounter. It makes you heal faster as well, so those wounds won't bother you so much for so long. This vitamin is highly favored & known for boosting your immune system.

Strengthens The Skin: Vitamin C boosts up collagen for you, which keeps your skin looking tight, elastic, & appearing vibrant for you. There are over 28 different types of collagen, the one that helps with your skin is type 4. It also prevents hyperpigmentation or dark spots on the skin & keeps your skin hydrated. You can get the most of these benefits through more topical use, but the diet you (plan to improve) will still reap these things for you!

Reduces high blood pressure & Improves heart health: According to the *Australia Stroke Foundation, "Blood pressure is a measure of the force with which blood presses on the walls of your arteries as it is pumped around your body..."*. Your blood pressure should be an average of 120/80, but if its 140/90, then you have high blood pressure or hypertension. High blood pressure is what causes strokes & damages the heart vessels. Hypertension'll also lead to heart diseases such as cardiomyopathy, which is when your heart becomes quite enlarged, to thicken or to have things that do NOT belong in the heart to be there, with (there are three types of cardiomyopathy). Vitamin C reduces the chances of these events occurring by reducing your cholesterol & reducing your blood pressure. While this is great news, please understand vitamin C alone will NOT make these problems go away, as a number of factors have to be introduced to assist in the reduction of these things happening, vitamin C is another tool to help you.

Too much Vitamin C

If you take in too much vitamin C, you'll start experiencing hair loss, fatigue, diarrhea, heartburn & insomnia. If that's not enough, you can experience rectum bleeding (you read that correctly), nose bleeding, muscle weakness & you'll be more irritable. Vitamin C is water soluble, so your body will rid the excess when you use the restroom, but don't think these things can't happen to, because they absolutely can.

Too little vitamin C

When your body doesn't all the vitamin C it needs, your wounds won't heal as fast, your gums become more susceptible to bleeding & swelling, you'll bruise more easily, your skin will be more dry & rough, & your joints will be more in pain. If you're to be deficient of vitamin C for a long period time, or chronically deficient, you'll develop an ailment known as scurvy, which can cause your gums to bleed or become purple, your skin to bleed underneath or a skin hemorrhage & very loose teeth that can fall out! You can cure this issue by eating plenty of vitamin C.

Foods rich in vitamin C

You can found an abundance of vitamin C in these foods: Strawberries, sweet potatoes, citrus fruits such as oranges, lemons, limes, tangerine & grapefruit. You can also look to Brussel sprouts, broccoli, kiwis, orange juice & chili peppers.

CHAPTER 9:

VITAMIN D (FAT SOLUBLE)

What is vitamin D (Calciferol)

Vitamin D is a vitamin that's important for the bones & teeth, brain & your immune system. As you may already know, being exposed to the sun triggers an alarm for the body to produce vitamin D, but how & why? When the ultraviolet rays from that huge star of ours hits our skin, a molecule in our skin known as 7-DHC is converted into vitamin pre-vitamin D through a strenuous chemical reaction & when your body is at the proper temperature or at least near, the benefits of vitamin D can last as long as three days! There's more on vitamin D, just continue on.

Benefits of Vitamin D

Calcium & Phosphorus absorption: Your bones need calcium & phosphorus to become stronger & vitamin D supports the absorption of these minerals. With stronger bones, you lower your chances of getting fractures of any type & studies have shown that vitamin D can even help with the preservation of muscle fibers. What that means is, your muscles are maintained well for your use & prolongs them!

Lowers chances of cancer: Studies have shown that vitamin D may be able to lower your chances of developing cancer, by slowing the progression of tumor cells & can even stop them from developing, especially for colon cancer. To this day though, more research is still needed, as the results from the tests haven't been steady.

Strengthens immune system: Vitamin D reduces inflammation within your body & activates white blood cells called lymphocytes or you may know them as 'T-cells'. These cells are what destroy infected cells & gives your body the protection against cancer cells. There are several types of T-cells which provides defense, suppression of pathogens & they can even remember previous infections for you! Go back to chapter 2 for more in depth of the white cells in general.

Prevents Diabetes: Diabetes, let it be one or two, is when the insulin in your body either isn't produced enough or is used incorrectly. It's also when your blood sugar levels are too high. With the help of Vitamin D & calcium, they'll stimulate your pancreas to secrete the insulin needed to function. Please note, vitamin D is not a sole solution to preventing/maintaining any type of diabetes.

Supports your skin: Vitamin D can help your skin by preventing aging & helps those out with eczema & psoriasis. If you don't have either of these issues, vitamin D prevents the development of acne as well.

Too much Vitamin D

When you take too much vitamin D, you'll experience something called hypercalcemia. Hypercalcemia is when you have too much calcium in your body & when it gets severe, you'll experience symptoms such as excessive urination. This is due to the fact that you're drinking a lot, thus making the kidneys work a whole lot harder than necessary, & all of that calcium can crystalized & become kidney stones. You'll also see your bones & muscles grow weaker because they're releasing too much calcium. Kind of ironic to say the least. On top of that, your blood pressure will skyrocket & your heartbeat rhythm will become abnormal.

Too little Vitamin D

When you're deficient in vitamin D, you'll go through mood changes, become fatigued & your joints will become painful, especially in your back. Your muscles will be weak & sore too. For adults, you may not even know you have a deficiency.

Food rich in vitamin D

You can found a lot of this vitamin in these foods: Almond milk, soy milk, yogurt, fish liver oil, dark chocolate, mushrooms, salmon & tuna.

CHAPTER 10:

VITAMIN E (FAT SOLUBLE)

What is vitamin E? (Tocopherol)

Vitamin E actually comes in eight forms of itself, but the form we need the most is called alpha-tocopherol. Its an antioxidant that fends off free radical, what we already explained in the previous chapter. It also improves your immune system, vision, blood & your brain, with other great perks. What's nice about this vitamin is that the daily intake isn't high like the other vitamins! (we'll get into that later on).

Benefits of vitamin E

Relieves Dysmenorrhea: Dysmenorrhea is extreme menstrual pain that's severe enough to affect daily life. These menstrual pains affect the same areas of a normal period of course. Vitamin E has been shown to reduce these pains & even more so when combined with omega-3 & vitamin C.

Relieves Oxidative stress: Vitamin E inserts its self in cell membranes to give the best defense against free radicals & it puts a holt to a process called 'lipid peroxidation'. To really understand lipid peroxidation, we need to know what lipids are. *Tolu Ajiboye* explained what lipids are best on the website *Verywell Health* by stating: *"Lipids are fatty, waxy, or oily compounds that are essential to many body functions and serve as the building blocks for all living cells. Lipids help regulate hormones, transmit nerve impulses, cushion organs, and store energy in the form of body fat."* There are three types of lipids, with triglyceride being most common within our bodies, gives us energy & guess what? They even aid in the absorption of fat soluble vitamins! Now when lipid peroxidation occurs, the free radicals attack the lipids within cells, leading to very bad cell damage & eventually, cell death. With vitamin E in the picture, it slows down the progression of new free radicals, destroys already existing ones & even promotes the repair of the cell membranes.

Supports eye health: Vitamin E has been linked to support your eyes & prevent the progression of Age-related Macular Degeneration (AMD). It really helps those who have already been diagnosed with this disease, by lowering the chances of it advancing by 25%. Vitamin E is to believed to have potential to aid against cataracts, which are formed by the oxidation of the lens of your eyes, especially by the sun. More research is needed to confirm these things though, as trials are still being performed to found consistent results.

Supports skin health: Vitamin E hasn't been proven to help with any serious ailments of the skin, however, it has been shown to aid against aging skin & helps with moisture , which is why it's found in many skin care products. Vitamin E is found in our skin oil (called sebum), giving our skins a protective barrier against bacteria & hydrates your skin. The lipids found in sebum is what gives the coating found on our skin. Sebum puts vitamin E on the surface of our skin, giving the protection needed to prevent damage of the skin. Along with this protection, vitamin E softens up your skin (via moisturizers), & can take in some UV rays from the sun (not all of it though, keep putting on your skin screen). Eating foods that contain vitamin E will help as well, & if you combine it with vitamin C, the benefits are amazing.

Reduces blood clots: Vitamin E foods have shown to reduce your chances of blood clotting in your heart. When blood clots take place in your heart, by blocking vessels & restricting blood flow, it'll result in a heart attack. Notice I said 'foods'. The supplements haven't shown any signs of reducing blood clots, the foods definitely have though.

It's also worth noting that the supplements haven't show to have much health benefits, in fact, its believed that increased dosage of vitamin E supplements can increase your chances of prostate cancer. More so, they haven't shown much improvement against Alzheimers, if at all. A healthy diet is always the best route.

Too much Vitamin E

If you take too much vitamin E, you'll experience some pretty serious side effects, such as a hemorrhagic stroke, a stroke that's triggered by your brain bleeding. Excessive vitamin E causes your blood to become thin, especially if you're already taking blood thinners. It can also disrupt blood clotting. Remember, blood clotting is your body's way of preventing excessive bleeding of any kind. Too much vitamin E can also interfere with cholesterol lowering medications & can interfere with cancer treatments as well, be sure to speak with a doctor about these things if your undergoing any treatments before taking in the supplements. Excessive vitamin E has also shown to disrupt the effects of vitamin K.

Too Little Vitamin E

When you're not getting the proper amount of vitamin E in your body, you'll face consequences that can be avoided. Your muscles will grow weaker & weaker, due to higher oxidative stress. Vitamin E is a very important vitamin for your body, both for the central nervous system & the immune system, your immune cells won't function properly without this vitamin. Your nervous system will suffer as well, your neurons are protected by mostly fat & when vitamin E doesn't have a strong presence within your body, it makes your neurons more susceptible to damage, causing your nervous system to deteriorate.

Foods rich in vitamin E

You can found this vitamin in these foods; potatoes, sunflower seeds, sunflower oil, mangoes, avocados, red bell peppers, hazel nut oil, snail, cray fish & lobster.

CHAPTER 11:

VITAMIN K (FAT SOLUBLE)

What is Vitamin K? (Phytonadione)

Vitamin K is a vitamin that plays a powerful role in strengthening your bones & support blood clot formation to aid in injury. This vitamin comes in a package a two, phylloquinone & menaquinone. To put in that in such an easier way, K1 & K2. Phylloquinone (filo-kwi-nohn) aka K1, is found mostly in plants & is the more common vitamin K, being consumed 75-90% of the time. The other vitamin K, menaquinone (men-ah-kwi-nohn) or K2, isn't as common & is found in some animal foods & fermented foods, with several subtypes existing! Both of the K's are needed to produce a protein called prothrombin, as its crucial for blood clots, bone metabolism & the health of your heart. The way both of these types are absorbed are different as well, so we'll look over the benefits. There's a third type of vitamin K, it's synthetic & is called menadione or K3, but is NOT safe for human consumption whatsoever, but seems safe for animals, so there will no consumption of vitamin K3 (as humans).

Benefits of vitamin K (both types)

Supports Bone Health: Vitamin K attaches to calcium, thus improving your bone density. K2 has been known to do this & in supplements, shown to lower your chances of bone fractures & support against osteoporosis, a disease that makes your bones weaker. Vitamin K activates a protein known as osteocalcin, it builds strong bones by binding to calcium & improving muscle strength.

Improves Blood Clotting: Vitamin K activates prothrombin, the protein apart of the process of blood clotting. Prothrombin changes into another compound called thrombin & then works with fibrin to start coagulating or clotting. These clots stop your bleeding injuries. Vitamin K also prevents your blood from being too thick or thin. Blood that's too thin will make you more prone to bruising & internal bleeding, while blood that's too thick will make you have increased blood pressure & dizziness. For women, thicker blood will cause prolonged menstrual bleeding.

Supports Blood Sugar: The protein osteocalcin, which is activated by vitamin K, not only helps with calcium & muscles, it also helps the pancreas secrete insulin into your cells. Insulin is a hormone that lets glucose (aka sugar) to get inside our cells, thus giving us energy. This vitamin is especially helpful for those with diabetes of either type. Type one diabetes is when no insulin or very little insulin is made, whilst type two diabetes is when insulin isn't used up completely.

Improves Heart Health: Vitamin K has been shown to stop calcium from building up within your heart, a process called 'calcification.' When calcium builds up in the arteries of the heart, it clogs them up with plaque. They build up in your coronary arteries, the two main arteries & restricts blood flow by piling up & making them more narrow. This'll cause chest pain & a heart attack for you. Some further studies are still needed to see if vitamin K can actually keep doing this though, even with some studies already showing it can do so.

Works with Vitamin D: Vitamin D also supports the absorption of calcium, so two vitamins doing this is a better bang for your buck! But there's a difference on how they do this. Vitamin K actually directs where the calcium goes within in the body, leading it to the right areas & preventing any health issues for you, while vitamin D improves your ability to absorb calcium. In essence, Vitamin D takes in calcium, while vitamin K tells it exactly where to go.

Essential for your infant: Newborn babies are deficient in vitamin K, even if the mother has a good amount of vitamin K in her body, very little is transferred to the baby via breastfeeding or if the mother has high levels if vitamin K. When the infant is deficient, they're more susceptible to severe bleeding. One time vitamin K injections have proven to be far more effective than oral vitamin K, since the oral supplement will have to be taken multiple time throughout time to even obtain the same benefits.

Too much vitamin K

Vitamin K toxicity is rare & in fact, hasn't been established for oral consumption, even in high amounts, but we'll go over why K3, aka menadione, isn't sold in supplements, especially since its more common for infants. When you have too much vitamin K in your body, you'll experience anemia through red blood cells rupturing & jaundice. Jaundice is when your skin & the white part of your eyes become yellow. Not only will your skin & eyes be yellow, your urine will also be very dark & your feces to be lighter It also disturbs the antioxidants in your body, causing oxidative stress. Vitamin K3 taking through injection has shown to cause liver damage. If you're taking blood thinners, vitamin K will decrease its effects as it supports blood clotting for you. Other than that, there really isn't too much on vitamin K toxicity, it's rare to say the least, as there's no established toxic level like the other vitamins.

Too little vitamin K

Believe it or not, most adults are vitamin K deficient. When you lack the proper amount of vitamin K you need, you'll go through things like excessive bleeding, when ever you get bruised or a cut, the bleeding is far more severe. You'll see blood in your feces or your urine. You'll bruise far more easily, along with dealing with bone fractures, as you have less bone density. Over time, you'll develop osteoporosis.

Foods rich in vitamin K

To get some vitamin K in your body, you can turn to these foods; blueberries, carrot juice, collared greens, broccoli, soybean oil, olive oil, spinach, pumpkin, lettuce, goose & beef livers, chicken, salami & grapes.

CHAPTER 12:

VITAMIN INTAKES A-B3

We went over every vitamin out there. We spoke on the benefits & drawbacks, now we need to discuss how much & how to take these vitamins. I said in the beginning that a diet is always the best way to get your vitamins in, but supplements are available as well. I want you to know that to receive the benefits of these vitamins, the diet is the best route. It's natural, delicious & fulfilling. Don't worry though, I'll discuss the supplements here as well, I had to get that out the way. Also, remember to discuss your health with your health care provider! There are conditions that can affect the way one can absorb & take in vitamins & minerals, so a diet alone may not help, & I am no doctor myself nor am I offering you medical advice. I'm giving insight of each vitamin & how they impact you as a human.

As you've read through this book, you learned how each vitamin may work in conjunction or may hinder one another. With these charts, you'll make informed decisions on your diet or supplements & you won't have to worry about vitamins cancelling each other out. With the assistance of a health care provider & your new (or refined) knowledge of these vitamins, rest assured, you'll be more than fine. We'll start the same routine over again, starting off with vitamin A & we'll work our way down the alphabet. This time, we'll go over how much of each vitamin you need to have a balanced diet & body. We'll also discuss the difference in the intakes of an actual diet & supplements. To make things better for you, all the foods listed out for each vitamin will be on here as well, showing how much of their respective vitamin they have. Some of these foods will be shown more than once, so don't be surprised or confused. Their servings will be shown as well, so how much of each vitamin you receive is also dependent on how much you eat, it should go without saying, that's NOT the only factor on how your body takes in these vitamins. Don't worry though, I'm going to take away all the confusion for you.

You'll be surprised by just how much vitamins some foods hold, don't roll your eyes at the measurements! This information will allow you to plan out meals more strategically. There are multiple ways food serving intakes are measured, but we'll just stick with the 'Recommended Daily Allowance' (RDA) chart to make things easy & show the 'Tolerable Upper Intake Level' (UL) to make sure you DO NOT enter the stages toxicity. The UL is the set max you can take before you experience toxicity, its tolerable, but once you go past those numbers, that's when the toxic effects kick in. We'll group up the vitamins for these parts as well. These amounts are whats considered safe for you day by day, to get an exact amount for yourself or child, go to the doctor & they'll gladly help you with that. Like the multitude of measurements of food, there are also different lists of higher & lower intakes, but again, we'll go with the RDA & UL. I'll be using websites called *'fat secret.com'* & *'NutritionIX'* to find these measurements & facts sheets for consumers & health professionals.

Finally, before continuing on, these established charts are set as standards for everyone. Remember, everyone is different, some may take medications & have conditions that may affect how much we need & how we take in these vitamins. It's imperative that you check in with a health care professional if you have any type of condition(s) or medications that can interfere with your vitamin absorptions. You may need less, you may need more, you may have to time things, you may not be able to take supplements or eat certain foods. Whatever the case may be, be sure to ask your doctor. This book can't replace your doctor's advice in any shape or form.

Vitamin A intake

To obtain the full benefits of retinol, it's recommended that adult men take in about 900 mcg (microgram)per day, women take in about 700 mcg per day, children ages 1-3 should take in about 300 mcg per day, children 4 -8 should take in 400 mcg per day, children 9-13 should take in 600 mcg per day, teenage boys ages 14-18 should take in about 900 mcg & teenage girls take in about 700 mcg. Pregnant teenage girls need about 750 mcg per day & if breastfeeding, need about 1,200 mcg. Adult women that are pregnant need about 770 mcg per day & if breastfeeding, need about

1,300 mcg per day. Infants ages 0-6 months need about 400 mcg per day & infants ages 7-12 months need 500 mcg per day.

To make sure you don't experience vitamin A toxicity (too much vitamin A) we have the UL listed out as well. Adults should not exceed 3,000 mcg per day (both men & women), children ages 1-3 shouldn't exceed 600 mcg per day & children 4-8 shouldn't exceed 900 mcg, children 9-13 shouldn't take in more than 1,700 mcg & teenagers ages 14-18 shouldn't exceed 2,800 mcg per day. Teenage girls & adult women that are pregnant shouldn't exceed 2,800 mcg per day & if breastfeeding, shouldn't exceed 3,000 mcg per day.

If you're taking any anti-coagulant drugs (anti blood clot), you may want to steer away from vitamin A supplements, as they'll increase your chances of bleeding. If you're taking retinoid drugs, including the topical cream, you're already receiving a high dosage of vitamin A, so taking in the supplements will make things bad for you. If you're taking tetracycline antibiotics & then take vitamin A supplements, you'll increase your chances of developing something known as intracranial hypertension, which is when the brain fluid pressure gets far too high & cause vision issues, even leading to blindness if left untreated & you'll feel dizzy & be more irritated. Intracranial hypertension can even cause death. To get a refresh of what vitamin A toxicity (or any other vitamins) are, run back through the pages to see what the symptoms are.

Now, on to the foods we've listed out for vitamin A, here they are & how much of vitamin A they have & their calorie count, measured in 1 oz serving:

Beef liver: 38 calories, 1,408 mcg of vitamin A

Lamb liver: 39 calories, 2,095 mcg of vitamin A

Boneless Salmon: 41 calories, 9mcg of vitamin A

Mangos: 18 calories, 11mcg of vitamin A

Carrots: 12 calories, 238mcg of vitamin A

Red peppers: 7 calories, 45mcg of vitamin A

Vitamin A supplements come in different forms & dosages. If you're buying over-the-counter supplements or prescribed some by a doctor, first listen to your doctor. for OTC, read the directions of that supplement & plan accordingly. I keep emphasizing that the diet is always better. If you have any conditions that inhibit your ability to absorb any vitamin, speak with your doctor about dosages & the form of them. I had to say that before continuing on.

Vitamin B1 intake

In order to get the necessary amount of thiamine running through your body, adult men need around 1.2 mcg per day, adult women need 1.1 mcg per day, children ages 1-3 need about 0.5 mcg per day, children ages 4-8 need 0.6 mcg per day, children ages 9-13 need around 0.9 mcg per day, teenage boys need about 1.2 mcg per day & teenage girls need about 1 mcg per day. Teenage girls & adult women that are pregnant & breastfeeding need about 1.4 mcg per day. Adult men ages 51+ need about 1.2 mcg & women ages 51+ need about 1.1 mcg per day. Infants ages 0-6 months 0.2 mcg & infants ages 7-12 months need about 0.3 mcg. As you can see, you don't need too much of this vitamin, a little bit goes a long way. Still important though, make sure to get this in your body! As stated when we went over B1, there's been no toxic limit set, but still do be careful & don't be the guinea pig for everyone else to find out! Since the recommended amount of B1 is so low, the 1 oz rate of measurement I had planned has to be put to the side to bring you the information you're seeking & need.

For our food list that was listed for B1, here's calorie count & amount of B1.

Pork chop: 158 calories, 0.4mcg of vitamin B1

Canned black beans: 218 calories, 0.4 mcg of vitamin B1, 1-1/2 cup

Trout: 172 calories, 0.4 mcg of vitamin B1, 3 oz

Egg noodles: 221 calories, 0.5 mcg of vitamin B1, 1 cup

Vitamin B1 supplements usually come in multivitamins or can be a sole vitamin. It's really helpful for those dealing with withdrawals of alcohol. Get some magnesium & your body will absorb this vitamin so much easier. Just like vitamin A (& all other vitamins) B1 supplements come in different dosages & forms.

Vitamin B2 Intake

For riboflavin, adult men need 1.3 mcg per day, adult women need 1.1 mcg per day, children ages 1-3 need 0.5 mcg per day, children ages 4-8 need 0.6 mcg per day, children ages 9-13 need 0.9 mcg per day, teenage boys need about 1.3 mcg per day & teenage girls need at least 1 mcg per day. Teenage girls & adult women that are pregnant need about 1.4 mcg per day & if breastfeeding, need about 1.6 mcg per day. Infants ages 0-6 months need about 0.3 mcg & infants ages 7-12 months need about 0.4 mcg. You'll start to notice a pattern based on vitamin B that they come in small amounts. There has been NO toxic level set for B2.

The food list for vitamin B2

Beef: 220 calories, 0.4 mcg of vitamin B2, 3 oz

Clams: 126 calories, 0.4 mcg of vitamin B2, 3 oz

Fat free yogurt: 95 calories, 0.6 mcg of vitamin B2, 6 oz

3 slices of Swiss cheese: 150 calories, 0.3 mcg of vitamin B2, 3 oz (each slice is 1 oz)

You can speak with your doctor about B2 supplements & found them the same way you can B1. All the B vitamins will be bunched in 'B-Complex' supplements.

Vitamin B3 Intake

Niacin intakes for adult men & teenage boys start at 16 mg (milligrams) per day, 14 mg for adult women & teenage girls, children ages 1-3 need 6 mg per day, children ages 4-8 need about 8 mg per day & children ages 9-13 need 12 mg per day. Infants ages 0-6 months need about 2 mg & infants ages 7-12 months need about 4 mg per day. Teenage girls & adult women that are pregnant need about 18 mg per day & if breastfeeding, need about 17 mg per day.

To avoid B3 toxicity, the UL established is as follows: For adult men & women, the limit is 35mg per day, children ages 1-3 is 10 mg per day, children ages 4-8 is 15 mg per day, children ages 9-13 is 20 mg per day & teenagers ages 14-18 is 30 mg per day. For teenage girls pregnant & breastfeeding, the limit is 30 mg per day. Adult women pregnant & breastfeeding, the limit is 35 mg per day.

Getting B3 from a diet is safe, but the supplements can causes health issues. When taking in a single dose between 30-50 mg or more, you'll experience niacin flush. That's when your skin becomes red, itchy, or a burning feeling. These effects can happen as quickly as 30 mins after intake or can happen within days of continuing to take these supplements. Throw in dizziness, low blood pressure & headaches in the mix as well. According to the *NIH,* you can lower the side effects by taking the supplements with food, slowly increasing your dosage intake overtime or you can wait for your body to become tolerant. Dosages of 1,000-3,000mg cause heartburn, fatigue, impaired vision, insulin resistance & something called macular edema, which is when your blood vessels are damaged & leak into the macula of the eye. The macula allows you to see details such as written words & with macular edema, the macula swells up, making colors look abnormal, making it a challenge to read anything & things can look wavy for you. If left untreated, it can cause severe vision loss & even blindness.

With all of that being said, let's take a look at the foods listed for vitamin B3.

Tuna: 111 calories, 8.6 mg of vitamin B3, 3 oz

Chicken Breast: 141 calories, 11.4 mg of vitamin B3, 3 oz

Peanut Butter: 188 calories, 4.3 mg of vitamin B3, 2 tablespoons

Mushrooms: 44 calories, 2.5 mg of vitamin B3, 1 cup

If you're consuming alcohol, taking in B3 supplements can worsen the symptoms of niacin flushing. B3 supplements can also make things worse for you if you're suffering from liver disease & can increase your blood sugar levels, especially if you have diabetes. Make sure to consult with your doctor about any concerns about niacin supplements.

CHAPTER 13:

B5-B12 INTAKES

Vitamin B5 intake

To make sure you get the proper amount of pantothenic acid in you, adult men & women need about 5mg per day, children ages 1-3 need about 2 mg per day, children ages 4-8 need about 3 mg per day & children ages 9-13 need about 4 mg per day. Teenage girls ages 14-18 that are pregnant & breastfeeding need about 6-7mg per day, the same being for adult women pregnant & breast feeding. Infants ages 0-6 months need 1.7 grams per day & infants ages 7-12 months need about 1.8 grams per day. Although there are no serious side effects to high dosages of B5 & no UL has been set, 10-20mg per day can cause diarrhea & other side effects mentioned.

AHere are the foods listed for B5.

Boiled broccoli: 27.5 calories, 0.5 mg of vitamin B5, 1/2 cup

Non-fat greek yogurt: 121.9 calories, 0.6 mg of vitamin B5, 5.3 oz

Canned chickpeas: 171 calories, 0.4 mg of vitamin B5, 1/2 cup

Mushrooms: 22 calories, 0.8 mg of vitamin B5, 1/2 cup

B5 supplements can interfere with the effectiveness of some antibiotic drugs & some Alzheimer's drugs as well, making them less potent for you. Always speak with your doctor before taking any supplements, especially if you're already on medications.

Vitamin B6 Intake

Pyridoxine RDA intakes for adult men & women is 1.3mg, children ages 1-3 is 0.5mg, children ages 4-8 is 0.6mg, children ages 9-13 is 1 mg, teenagers ages 14-18 need 1.2-1.3mg per day, teenage girls ages 14-18 & adult women that are pregnant & breastfeeding need 1.9-2mg per day& adult men 51 years or older need about 1.7, adult women 51 years or older need about 1.5 mg. Infants ages 0-6 months need 0.1 mg per day & infants ages 7-12 months need 0.3mg per day. We went over the toxicity of B6 in chapter 7, which includes neuropathy & sensory ataxia, which mostly stem from (but not limited to) the supplements.

To avoid toxicity, the established UL for adult men & women is 100 mg per day, children ages 1-3 is 30 mg per day, children ages 4-8 is about 40 mg per day, children ages 9-13 is about 60 mg per day, teenagers ages 14-18 is about 80 mg per day, teenage girls pregnant & breastfeeding is about 80 mg per day & adult women pregnant & breastfeeding is 100 mg per day.

The food list for B6.

Chicken breast: 141 calories, 0.5 mg of vitamin B6, 3 oz

Plain waffles: 218 calories, 0.3 mg of vitamin B6, 1 waffle

Salmon: 174 calories, 0.6 mg of vitamin B6, 3 oz

Boiled potatoes: 166 calories, 0.4 mg of vitamin B6, 1 cup

There are medicines that can interfere with the level of vitamin B6 in your body, such as seizure medicines, cancer medicines, & tuberculosis treatments. Vitamin B6 itself can lower the effectiveness of Levodopa, a medicine used to treat Parkinson's disease. Make sure to consult with your doctor before taking any supplements, especially if you're already on medications.

Vitamin B7 Intake

Moving on to Biotin, the necessary intakes for adult men & women is 30 mcg per day, children ages 1-3 is 8 mcg per day, children ages 4-8 is 12 mcg per day, children ages 9-13 need 20 mcg per day, & teenagers ages 14-18 is 25 mcg per day Infants ages 0-6 months need 5mcg & infants ages 7-12 months need about 6 mcg. Teenage girls & adult women that are pregnant need 30 mcg per day & if breastfeeding, need 35 mcg per day. Despite no UL being set for this vitamin, a high dosage of vitamin B7 will cause lab results for medical tests such as for thyroid tests, to be false & misleading. When you have false lab readings, that's detrimental to your health & even your life, because you have an improper diagnosis!

The food list for vitamin B7.

Pink Salmon: 174 calories, 5.0 mcg of vitamin B7, 3 oz

Sweet potato: 154.5 calories, 2.4 mcg of vitamin B7, 1/2 cup

Bananas: 250.5 calories, 0.2 mcg of vitamin B7, 1/2 cup

Eggs: 72 calories, 10 mcg of vitamin B7, whole egg

Anti seizure medicines have shown to lower biotin levels, due to the fact that some anti seizure medications interfere with the absorption of biotin. Speak with your doctor about taking supplements if you're on medications.

Vitamin B9 Intake

Folate intakes for adult men & women is 400 mcg per day, children ages 1-3 is 150 mcg per day , children ages 4-8 is 200 mcg per day & children ages 9-13 is 300 mcg per day. When you have high dosages of vitamin B9, not only does it hide vitamin B12 deficiency, but you won't know about it until you start suffering from brain damage from the lack of B12. high dosages of folic acid can also reduce the amount of white cells in your body, which is what we don't want for our immune system.

To avoid B9 toxicity, adult men & women should never go pass 1,000 mcg per day, children ages 1-3 should never exceed 300 mcg per day, children ages 4-8 should never exceed 400 mcg per day, children ages 9-13 should never exceed 600 mcg per day & teenagers ages 14-18 should never exceed 800 mcg per day. Pregnant & breastfeeding teenage girls should never exceed 800 mcg & adult women pregnant & breastfeeding should never exceed 1,000 mcg per day. No UL for infants has been established due to formula, breast milk & food being the only necessary sources for them.

The foods listed for vitamins B9.

Asparagus: 13 calories, 89 mcg of vitamin B9, 4 spears

Bananas: 105 calories, 24 mcg of vitamin B9, 1 medium banana

Beef liver: 162 calories, 215 mcg of vitamin B9, 3 oz

Tomato juice: 31 calories, 36 mcg of vitamin B9, 3/4 cup

A drug known as sulfasalazine is used to treat ulcerative colitis, which is an inflammatory bowel disease that causes sores (the ulcers) & inflames your digestion system. Sulfasalazine can reduce your body's ability to absorb vitamin B9, causing a deficiency. Anti epileptic medications can reduce folate serums as well. Speak with a doctor about B9 supplements.

Vitamin B12 Intake

To receive the proper amount of cobalamin, adult men & women need about need about 2.4 mcg per day, children ages between 1-3 need about 0.9 mcg per day, children ages between 4-8 need about 1.2 mcg per day, children ages 9-13 need about 1.8 mcg per day & teenagers ages 14-18 need about 2.4 mcg per day. Pregnant & breast feeding teenage girls & adult women need 2.6-2.8 mcg per day. Infants ages 0-6 months 0.4 mcg per day & infants ages 7-12 months need about 0.5 mcg per day. While there is no toxic level establish for vitamin B12, the supplements is where concern can begin.

A look at the foods rich in vitamin B12.

Fat free plain yogurt: 95 calories, 1 mcg of vitamin B12, 6 0z

Soy milk: 100 calories, 2.07 mcg of vitamin B12, 1 cup

Grilled steak: 614 calories, 11.2 mcg of vitamin B12, 1 steak

Salmon: 174 calories, 2.6 mcg of vitamin B12, 3 oz

Vitamin B12 in supplement format has NO effect on endurance or performance whatsoever. Supplements of vitamin B12 by itself or in combination with other B vitamins or B-complex has no capability of preventing heart attacks nor can it lower the chance of death for those suffering from cardiovascular disease. A medicine known as metformin, which treats pre diabetes & diabetes, could reduce your body's ability to absorb B12, along with gastric inhibitors, which slow down gastric acid release, causing a B12 deficiency. Speak with your doctor about taking B12 supplements before taking them.

CHAPTER 14:

C-K INTAKES

Vitamin C Intake

Ascorbic acid intake levels for adult men is 90 mg per day, adult women is 75 mg per day, children ages 1-3 is about 15 mg per day , children ages 4-8 is about 25 mg per day, children ages 9-13 require about 75 mg per day, teenage boys ages 14-18 need about 75mg per day & teenage girls need about 65 mg per day. Pregnant women need about 85mg per day & breastfeeding women need about 120 mg per day. Infants ages 0-6 months need about 40 mg per day & infants ages 7-12 months need about 50 mg per day. Due to the oxidative stress created when smoking, those who are habitual smokers need 35 mg more per day & if you're exposed to second hand smoke, you may want to make sure to increase your intakes as well. Be wary of feeding infants heated milk or cow milk, as cow milk isn't high enough in vitamin C & heat destroys vitamin C.

To make sure you avoid toxic levels of vitamin C, the UL established for adult men & women shouldn't exceed 2,000mg per day, children ages 1-3 should avoid exceeding 400 mg per day, children ages 4-8 should avoid exceeding 650 mg per day, children ages 9-13 should avoid exceeding 1,200mg per day, & teenagers ages 14-18 shouldn't exceed 1,800 mg per day. Teenage girls ages 14-18 that pregnant & breastfeeding should avoid exceeding 1,800 mg. Adult women pregnant & breastfeeding should avoid exceeding 2,000 mg. No UL has been established for infants due to formula & food being the only sources necessary for them.

The foods listed for vitamin C.

Strawberries: 56 calories, 49 mg of vitamin C, 1/2 cup

Brussel sprouts: 28 calories, 48 mg of vitamin C, 1/2 cup

Kiwi: 55 calories, 64 mg of vitamin C, 1/2 cup

Orange juice: 78.4 calories, 93 mg of vitamin C, 3/4 cup

If you're on chemotherapy drugs, vitamin C supplements can reduce their effectiveness due to some studies suggesting they protect tumor cells. These studies have been criticized however, by some doctors suggesting the supplements may protect normal tissues. Due to these conflicting studies & more research needed, it's best to speak with your doctor if on chemotherapy.

Vitamin D Intake

To make sure you get the right amount of calciferol into your body, adult men & women, teenage boys & girls, ages 13-70 need about 15 mcg per day. The same amount of 15 mcg per day is required for children ages 1-12 as well. Adults ages 70 & older will need about 20 mcg per day. Pregnant & breastfeeding women need about 15 mcg per day. Infants ages 0-12 months need about 10 mcg per day. Every individual will have different intake requirements, which are affected by sun exposure, the latitude you live upon, obesity, age & skin tone.

To avoid vitamin D toxicity, adult men & women & teenage boys & girls should never go exceed 100 mcg per day (13-70+), children ages 9-12 shouldn't exceed 100 mcg per day, children ages 4-8 shouldn't exceed 75 mcg per day & children ages 1-3 shouldn't exceed 63 mcg per day. Pregnant & breastfeeding women shouldn't exceed 100 mcg. Infants ages 0-6 months shouldn't exceed 25 mcg & infants ages 7-12 months shouldn't exceed 38 mcg.

The foods listed for vitamin D.

Almond milk: 56 calories, 2.5-3.6 mcg, 1 cup

Soy milk: 100 calories, 2.92 mcg, 1 cup

Cod liver oil: 122 calories, 34 mcg, 1 tablespoon

Mushrooms: 22 calories, 9.2 mcg, 1/2 cup

You can leave mushrooms in the sun for 15-20 mintues & they'll have even higher levels of vitamin D. Steroid medications used to reduce inflammation disrupt the absorption of calcium & vitamin D, along with a weight loss drug called Orlistat, can also reduce vitamin D absorption. If you're taking any medications, especially ones mentioned, be sure to speak with your doctor before taking vitamin D supplements.

Vitamin E Intake

The RDA for tocopherol intakes for ages 14 & up for both men & women is 15 mg per day, children ages 1-3 need about 6 mg per day, children ages 4-8 need about 7 mg per day & children ages 9-13 need about 11 mg per day. Teenage girls & women pregnant & breastfeeding need about 15 mg per day, infants 0-6 months need about 4 mcg per day & infants 6-12 months need about 5 mcg per day.

To make sure you don't go into vitamin E toxicity, adult men & women shouldn't exceed 1,000 mg per day, children ages 1-3 shouldn't exceed 200 mg per day, children ages 4-8 shouldn't exceed 300 mg per day, children ages 9-13 shouldn't exceed 600 mg per day & teenagers ages 14-18 shouldn't exceed 800 mg. Pregnant & breastfeeding women ages 14-18 shouldn't exceed 800 mg & adult women pregnant & breastfeeding shouldn't exceed 1,000 mg per day.

The foods listed for vitamin E.

Sunflower oil: 121 calories, 5.6 mg of vitamin E, 1 tablespoon

Sunflower seeds: 155 calories, 7.4 mg of vitamin E, 1 tablespoon

Snail: 26 calories, 1.4 mg of vitamin E, 1 oz

Red sweet pepper: 37 calories, 1.9 mg of vitamin E, 1 medium pepper

Vitamin E supplements have shown to reduce the effectiveness of chemotherapy medications by preventing them from destroying cancerous cells, though more research is needed to find more information about the relations of vitamin E supplements & chemotherapy medicines. Vitamin E has also shown to increase your chances of prostate cancer, when it was believed to reduce your chances. Researchers aren't sure why that is, but tell patients to be cautious of the supplements, with some conflicting studies saying it can help, even with little effect. Do not take any vitamin E supplements in the first 8 weeks of pregnancy, as this'll cause issues for the baby. Be sure to speak with your doctor before taking vitamin E supplements.

Vitamin K Intake

The recommended RDA for phytonadione for adult men is 120mcg per day, adult women 90 mcg per day, children ages 1-3 is 30 mcg per day, children ages 4-8 is 55 mcg per day, children ages 9-13 is 60 mcg per day, & teenagers ages 14-18 is 75 mcg per day. Pregnant & breastfeeding adult women need about 90 mcg per day & pregnant & breastfeeding teenager is 75 mcg per day. Infants 0-6 months need 2 mcg per day & infants 7-12 months need about 2.5 mcg per day.

There's no established UL for vitamin K & we discussed the dangers of vitamin K3, don't even worry about running across it in your favorite store, it's banned from being sold (to humans at least).

The foods we have for vitamin K.

Olive oil: 119 calories, 8mcg of vitamin K, 1 tablespoon

Soybean oil: 104 calories, 25 mcg of vitamin K, 1 tablespoon

Blueberries: 42 calories, 14 mcg of vitamin K, 1/2 cup

Spinach: 41 calories, 145 mcg of vitamin K, 1 cup

Grapes: 52 calories, 11 mcg of vitamin K, 1/2 cup

Antibiotics destroy the bacteria that produce vitamin K in the gut, decreasing vitamin K levels & even restricting activity of vitamin K. However, this usually won't be an issue unless taking antibiotics for long periods of time & you have low vitamin K intake.

CHAPTER 15:

SOME MINERALS

We brought up some minerals that compliment our vitamins, so it only makes sense to discuss those minerals & some unmentioned. I'll give some brief descriptions of some minerals & what foods you can found them in.

Calcium- The most abundant mineral within your body, it does more than give you healthy bones & teeth as it's widely known for. It also helps out with blood clotting, supports muscle contraction (stretching, lifting, holding things etc) & supports your nerve system. Vitamin D can help your body absorb this mineral a whole lot better.

You can found loads of calcium in almonds, soy milk, chia seeds, tofu & cheese

Phosphorus- The 2nd most abundant mineral within your body, you'll find it as it's salted version, phosphate, in the body, so you wouldn't be wrong to say either term, especially if taken as a supplement. Like calcium, it helps with building & maintaining your bones. It also helps with your metabolism, your normal heart beat, DNA, RNA & ATP. It also makes sure your blood's pH level is where it's suppose to be.

You can found a good amount of phosphorus in beef, sunflower seeds, chicken, pinto beans & whole wheat bread.

Iron- You need iron because it creates the hemoglobin within your red blood cells & that allows oxygen to be transported into your blood & throughout your body. This transported oxygen is what allows you to have high energy for anything you do & gives you better focus as well. Pregnant women will need a surplus of iron to support a literal human inside of them. There are two types of iron; heme, which is found in animal foods & non-heme, which is found in plants. Your body absorbs heme-iron much better. Calcium can actually hinder the absorption of iron all around, so be sure to eat foods rich in vitamin A & D, it's also recommended to not take iron & calcium supplements at the same time.

Foods rich in iron are strawberries, citrus fruits, raisins, beef & chicken.

Zinc- This mineral helps with your immune system, & your metabolism. Zinc has shown to lower blood sugar & lower cholesterol, especially for those with type 2 diabetes. It also lowers your chances of developing AMD (see vitamin E) & expedites healing from a cold. The topical ointment of zinc, called 'zinc-oxide' or even the supplement of it, can heal wounds faster & improves the health of sperms & supports fetal health. Too much of zinc can interfere with the absorption of copper & magnesium. Calcium supplements can interfere with zinc absorption.

Foods rich in zinc are oysters, dark chocolate, beef, lamb & pork

Copper- Copper helps with the formation of white blood cells, supports brain health, reduce free radical population & supports the formation of collagen. Copper also works side-by-side with melanin in your body, makes sure your skin is healthy & along with other antioxidants, slows skin aging. Along side iron, it also helps with the formation of red blood cells.

You can found copper abundantly in these foods: Salmon, avocado, oyster, sunflower seeds & black pepper.

Magnesium- Over 68% of Americans are deficient in magnesium & with it being the 4th most abundant mineral in your body & playing a very important role, it's unfortunate to say the least. Magnesium helps with memory & learning in the brain, builds DNA, helps control your blood sugar, blood pressure & it helps makes sure your heartbeat is normal & properly with the aid of calcium. It helps with the formation & strengthening of yor bones, just like calcium. You see, calcium makes muscle fibers for your heart to contract, whilst magnesium helps your heart to relax. It goes beyond your heart, it allows the rest of your muscles to relax with calcium stimulates them. They counter one another as you can see, but in a good way. It's why magnesium is given to those with muscle cramps & spams to aid in the healing. You see, magnesium & calcium complement each other so well that if taken together, you boost both of their benefits. Magnesium allows you to sleep better at night, which a lot of people struggle with, though more research will be needed.

These foods are rich with magnesium: pumpkin seeds, almonds, peanut butter, soy milk, bananas & dark chocolate

Potassium- The 3rd most bounteous mineral in the body, it's highly reactive in water, to where it's considered an electrolyte once inside the system because it can conduct electricity, making it perfect to support nerve signaling. It helps with muscle contractions, regulate bodily fluids, takes waste out of your cells, & puts nutrients & water into your cells. It reduces the negative imprint of sodium & relieves blood vessel walls, helping you with blood pressure.

High levels of potassium can be found in these foods: bananas, watermelons, coconut water, pomegranates & spinach

Sodium- You may know sodium by its other name, 'salt'. You know, the salt you use for your fries & the ones you see at your grocery store? It's practically found in everything you consume whether its naturally there or its processed into those bag of chips in your pantry, it's no surprise that sodium is constantly disparaged & slandered & for good reason to be honest. All the health risks that come with it such as strokes, clogged arteries, high blood pressure etc. makes it seem like such an evil mineral. But let's realistic, too much of *anything* is bad for you, obviously. Sodium is an electrolyte that your body needs, believe it or not. It controls blood volume & fluid around cells. It also allows normal functionality of your nerves & muscles. Sodium also allows your brain to function up to its peak performance, removes excess carbon dioxide & keeps your hydrated. Get this, sodium actually maintains your blood pressure! It keeps your heart contractions stable, when it's in excess, it shoots up your blood pressure & that in itself is a problem. There's quite a debate on how much to consume sodium, as different health agencies have established different RDAs, & not everyone has the same reaction to sodium either, so its best to speak to your doctor to see what you need.

The foods that sodium comes in: Cottage cheese, soy sauce, olives, pickles, ketchup, mustard, potato fries & croutons.

CHAPTER 16:

YOUR NEW KNOWLEDGE

You made it this far into the book & with your newly acquired knowledge, you're better equipped to a healthier lifestyle! Please understand, like everything else in the world, there are new discoveries, debunked myths, established laws etc. With that being said, the information presented to you in this book is as accurate as possible, made simple & clear for your benefit & done so with making absolute sure the information is correct.

Your health goes beyond vitamins & minerals as well. You have to dedicate yourself to exercise, life changes, make or break habits. I've listed foods to help you out but those listed foods are not the *only* foods that contain such vitamins & minerals. There's a plethora of food choices for you to choose from. I encourage you, the reader, to do more research & gain more knowledge to make sure you & the ones you consider close to you, become healthier & better.

I've learned quite a lot myself while writing this book & I'm so glad that I was able to help you out in your journey to being more healthy. To help you means a lot to me, knowing I did something good for someone else makes the writing of this book worth it. Good luck on your goals & stick to your plans, no matter what.

Made in the USA
Columbia, SC
13 March 2025